Optimized Nutrition

MINIMUM CALORIES, MAXIMUM NUTRITION

A 7-day meal plan by Mark Raymond

Copyright 2017

ACKNOWLEDGEMENTS

Thanks to the many people and organizations who have inspired me over the years to improve my nutrition, increase my level of fitness, and optimize my overall well-being:

Elizabeth Quigley, Registered Dietitian
College of The Desert, Adjunct faculty

Kris Gunnars, Authority Nutrition
healthline.com/nutrition

CRON-O-Meter
cronometer.com

Tyler Graham and Drew Ramsey, MD
Authors of *The Happiness Diet*

Emeran Mayer, MD
Author of *The Mind-Gut Connection*

Jean Pierre Fux
Certified Personal Trainer

Gallup-Sharecare Well-Being Index
well-beingindex.com

And my dear mother, Jan

A special thanks to Kris Gunnars: His fantastic meal plans from *Authority Nutrition* inspired many of the recipes in this book. His meal plan service is now defunct, sadly, but I will continue to use and adapt his delicious and nutritious recipes for many years to come.

Optimized Nutrition
A 7-Day Meal Plan Based on Real Food

How's your diet? Are you getting the vitamins and minerals you need through food alone, or do you take daily supplements to help fill in the gaps? If you're taking supplements, how much do you need to take? If you have no idea, this guide is a good place to start. In it, you'll find a 7-day meal plan based on vitamin and mineral recommendations from the USDA for the average American. The guidelines are based on a 2000-calorie daily diet.

A few notes before we get started:

WATER

In order to meet the daily nutritional goals, you should drink at least 8 cups of water. This is not as difficult as some would believe. Often, we hear that we should drink "8 glasses of water" per day. This advice probably started with the advice to drink 8 cups of water, but then evolved into "8 glasses". A typical beverage glass in the US has a 16-ounce capacity – that's two cups. If you drank 8 glasses, that would be 16 cups of water per day, which is truly unnecessary. Don't torture yourself trying to consume enough water. Eight cups per day is plenty for most of us. I like to make it relatively easy on myself by drinking water throughout the day to ensure I get enough.

Since the meal plan is structured around eating five meals per day, my suggestion for water intake is the following:

>   2 cups with breakfast
>
>   1 cup with snack #1
>
>   2 cups with lunch
>
>   1 cup with snack #2
>
>   2 cups with dinner

If you're also drinking water while exercising or working, great! You have even less to think about. You may also count the water you consume in other drinks such as tea, or in the soups you make.

The reason for drinking water is not simply for hydration. Water also contains important micronutrients such as calcium, copper, magnesium, and zinc. I factor this into the nutritional summaries at the end of each day's meals. So, to meet the nutritional goals, you must drink your water.

MEASUREMENTS

The nutritional analyses I've provided are based on precise measurements of ingredients for each recipe. I do provide common measurements for those who take a more casual approach, but I highly recommend buying a small digital scale to weigh your ingredients. Doing this ensures that your nutritional intake will be more accurate. It's also a cleaner style of cooking; adding ingredients to a bowl on a scale creates less of a mess than using individual measuring cups - which then have to be cleaned later.

VITAMIN D

I do not include nutritional targets for Vitamin D, primarily because it can be a real challenge to get the Vitamin D you need through food alone. In recent years, getting tested for Vitamin D has become popular. Recent news suggests, however, that this is not necessary, and in fact, Vitamin D supplements (like many other supplements) can bring their own set of problems. If you're truly concerned about your Vitamin D levels, talk with your doctor or dietician. Otherwise, just spend some time out in the sun every day – 10 or 15 minutes a day is usually enough. Since I include a healthy amount of eggs and dairy foods in my meal plan, you'll be sure to get at least a fair amount of Vitamin D every day, even if you don't venture out into the sun for long.

ORGANIC AND GRASS-FED DAIRY FOOD

If you truly want to optimize your nutrition, I recommend buying organic foods and grass-fed dairy foods whenever possible. If it's beyond what your budget allows, don't put yourself in debt for it, but you should always try to eat foods that are natural and high in quality.

INGREDIENTS

It's almost a cliché now, but if the list of ingredients on a package of foods includes ingredients that you don't recognize, you may want to think twice about eating it. Get used to reading ingredient lists, and look up those that you don't recognize.

SWEETENERS

Avoid sugar and artificial sweeteners. The good news is that there are natural sweeteners, such as honey, real maple syrup, and molasses, which all have small but useful amounts of micronutrients that our bodies need. Sugar and artificial sweeteners contain none of these. In fact, artificial sweeteners are possibly even worse than sugar: Studies show that artificial sweeteners can make our bodies absorb even more of the calories we eat, leading to weight gain. Just say no.

PROCESSED FOOD

It's an overused term: processed food. But is processed food necessarily bad? No, it is not. But again, you want to think about where the food came from, and how it was manufactured. An easy rule to follow: If nature made the food you're about to eat, it's probably okay; if the food was created in a chemistry lab, beware. The bottom line? Eat real food.

TRACKING YOUR OWN NUTRITION

I strongly recommend using a nutrient-tracking app such as Cronometer. There are many macronutrient trackers on the market, but Cronometer is the only one I know of that also tracks vitamins and minerals. It's essential in making the most of your diet and nutrition.

Daily Dietary Goals

The following tables show you the recommended macro- and micronutrient goals that I use in this guide. The recommendations come from the USDA's Dietary Guidelines, which are based on a dietary intake of 2000 calories per day. You'll see the tables at the end of each recipe, as well as a nutritional summary at the end of each day's meals.

Although nutritional goals are set for most values, I have chosen to not set any minimum or maximum goals for carbohydrates or fat. The reasons are twofold: 1) Unless you are on an unusual diet, you will easily satisfy the minimum recommended intakes for carbohydrates and fat, and 2) Research shows that, in terms of losing weight and body fat, dietary macronutrient composition is irrelevant (or at the very least, nearly irrelevant). For most people, as long as you don't have any metabolic disorders (such as diabetes), the fundamentals of effective weight loss are simply a matter of reducing your calorie intake. I know that doesn't sound very exciting in this age of low-carb everything, but it's true: In order to lose weight and body fat, you must burn more energy (in the form of calories) than you consume. Fad diets be damned!

All vitamin and mineral goals are minimum amounts to be met every day. No maximums are set, except for sodium. A maximum of 2300 mg of sodium is typically recommended for optimal health. Although there is some ongoing debate in the medical and dietetic community about the optimal amount of dietary sodium, I think it's wise to be conservative about it until we know more. You'll find, however, that if you buy foods without sodium added by the manufacturer, adding your own sodium (preferably in the form of Himalayan sea salt, which also provides a healthy dose of iron) will give you more than enough to enhance the flavor of your foods.

Following the charts, you'll find Day One of the meal planner. I hope you'll find this guide both interesting and enjoyable to use. Have fun eating well as you optimize your nutrition!

Energy and Macronutrient Minimum Goals

	Amount
Calories	2000 (maximum)
Protein	50 g
Carbohydrates	No minimum/maximum
Fiber	28 g
Fat	No minimum/maximum
Omega-3 Fatty Acids	1.6 g

Daily Dietary Minimum Goals
Vitamin and Minerals

Vitamins

	Amount
Vitamin A (as Retinol Equivalent Activity)	900 µg
Vitamin B1 (Thiamine)	1.2 mg
Vitamin B2 (Riboflavin)	1.3 mg
Vitamin B3 (Niacin)	16 mg
Vitamin B5 (Pantothenic Acid)	5 mg
Vitamin B6 (Pyridoxine)	1.7 mg
Vitamin B9 (Folate)	400 µg
Vitamin B12 (Cobalamin)	2.4 µg
Vitamin C (Ascorbic Acid)	90 mg
Vitamin E (Tocopherol)	15 mg
Vitamin K (Phylloquinone)	120 µg
Choline	550 mg

Minerals

	Amount
Calcium	1300 mg
Copper	0.9 mg
Iron	18 mg
Magnesium	420 mg
Manganese	2.3 mg
Phosphorus	1250 mg
Potassium	4700 mg
Selenium	55 µg
Sodium	1500 mg
Zinc	11 mg

Your Shopping List

Check your pantry - you may have some of these already at home.

Dairy

Blue Cheese, crumbled (2 tablespoons)
Cottage cheese, fat-free (2 cups / 16 oz)
Eggs (12)
Feta cheese, reduced fat (1/2 cup)
Gorgonzola cheese, crumbled (2 tablespoons)
Milk, skim (1/2 gallon)
Mozzarella cheese, part skim, shredded (3/4 cup)
Parmesan cheese (2 tablespoons)
Sour cream, fat-free (2 tablespoons)
Yogurt, plain, fat-free (3 cups / 24 oz)

Vegetables

Arugula (15 leaves)
Baby carrots (67)

Barley, dry (2/3 cup)
Black beans, canned, low sodium (1 can / 14 oz)
Black olives (1 can / 16 oz)
Broccoli, raw (1 cup / 8 oz)
Carrots (2 medium)
Cucumber (1/4 medium)
Grape tomatoes (26)
Kale, frozen, chopped (1/4 cup / 2 oz)

Lentils, pink or red (2/3 cup / 6 oz)
Mushrooms, raw (1 cup / 8 oz)
Potato (1 large)
Red bell pepper (3/4 medium)
Red onion, medium (1/2)
Romaine lettuce (1½ cups)
Spinach, frozen (1½ cups / 12 oz)
Sweet potatoes (2 medium)
White or yellow onion (3)
Yellow bell pepper (1/2 medium)
Zucchini (1/2 small)

Fruits

Apple (1 small)
Apricots, dried (3)
Avocado (1)
Bananas (2 small, 2 medium, 1 large)
Blackberries, frozen, unsweetened (3/4 cup)
Blueberries, frozen, unsweetened (1/4 cup)
Cantaloupe (1/4 small)
Figs, dried (3)
Orange (1 small, 1 medium)
Pear (1 medium)
Raisins (1 tablespoon)
Strawberries (7)

Meats

Beef, ground, 75% lean (22½ oz)
Chicken breasts, boneless, skinless (4)
Clams, chopped (1 can / 6 oz)
Salmon, Wild Atlantic (10 oz)
Tuna, water pack (1 can)
Turkey, ground, lean, 7% fat (2½ oz)

Grains, seeds, nuts

Brown rice (3/4 cup / 6 oz)
Chia seeds (2/3 cup / 5 oz)
Flax seeds (1 tablespoon)
Oats, dry (3/4 cup / 6 oz)
Pumpkin seeds, shelled, unsalted (1 tablespoon)
Sunflower seeds, unsalted (1/4 cup)
Walnuts, chopped (2 tablespoons)
Whole wheat bread, thin-sliced (8)

Condiments, oils, spices

Blackstrap molasses (1/2 teaspoon)
Coconut oil (1/2 tablespoons)
Garlic cloves (5)
Himalayan sea salt (1/2 cup)
Honey (1½ tablespoons)
Lemon juice (2 tablespoons)
Maple syrup (1/2 teaspoon)
Olive oil (1/2 cup / 4 oz)
Oregano (2 tablespoons)
Poultry seasoning (2 tablespoons)
Red pesto sauce (2 tablespoons)
Salad dressing of your choice
Soy sauce, low sodium (1 teaspoon)
Thyme (1 tablespoon)

Other

Almond butter, unsalted (2 tablespoons)
Cocoa powder, unsweetened (2 teaspoons)
Dark chocolate chips, 70-85% cacao (1 tablespoon)
Dark chocolate bar, 70-85% cacao (1/4)
Tomato paste (2 tablespoons)
Tomato puree, sodium-free (3 cups)
Vegetable cooking stock (3 cups)

Day One

Breakfast
Avocado Toast with Cheesy Coconut Eggs

Snack #1
Blueberry Chocolate Chip Chia Honey Yogurt

Lunch
Black Bean Turkey Salad with Sunflower Seeds

Snack #2
Pear with Molasses Walnut Yogurt

Dinner
Beef Vegetable Lasagna with Whole Grain Bread

Avocado Toast with Cheesy Coconut Eggs
Day 1 - Breakfast

Ingredients	Weight
½ tablespoon coconut oil	7 g
¼ yellow bell pepper	30 g
½ cup chopped mushrooms	35 g
2 large eggs	100 g
$^{1}/_{16}$ teaspoon Himalayan sea salt	
3 tablespoons shredded reduced fat cheddar cheese	25 g
¼ avocado	34 g
2 thin slices whole wheat bread	48 g

Instructions:

1. Heat coconut oil in a medium skillet.
2. Sauté bell pepper and mushrooms for 3-4 minutes.
3. Whisk eggs and salt together in a bowl, then add to skillet.
4. While eggs are cooking, toast 2 slices of bread.
5. Add cheese and avocado to eggs and vegetables. Continue to cook until eggs are done, and cheese has melted.
6. Place slices of toast on a plate and spread the cooked egg mixture over the toast.

Energy and Macronutrient Summary

	Amount	Daily Value
Calories	488.2	24%
Protein	27.4 g	55%
Carbohydrates	28.6 g	
Fiber	5.8 g	21%
Fat	29.7 g	
Omega-3 Fatty Acids	0.2 g	12%

Avocado Toast with Cheesy Coconut Eggs
Vitamin and Mineral Analysis

Vitamins

	Amount	Daily Value
Vitamin A (as Retinol Equivalent Activity)	192.7 µg	21%
Vitamin B1 (Thiamine)	0.3 mg	27%
Vitamin B2 (Riboflavin)	0.9 mg	68%
Vitamin B3 (Niacin)	4.4 mg	28%
Vitamin B5 (Pantothenic Acid)	2.9 mg	58%
Vitamin B6 (Pyridoxine)	0.4 mg	25%
Vitamin B9 (Folate)	113.2 µg	28%
Vitamin B12 (Cobalamin)	1.5 µg	62%
Vitamin C (Ascorbic Acid)	58.8 mg	65%
Vitamin E (Tocopherol)	3.2 mg	21%
Vitamin K (Phylloquinone)	12.3 µg	10%
Choline	323.3 mg	59%

Minerals

	Amount	Daily Value
Calcium	327.1 mg	25%
Copper	0.3 mg	37%
Iron	3.3 mg	18%
Magnesium	69.4 mg	17%
Manganese	1.2 mg	51%
Phosphorus	459.4 mg	37%
Potassium	613.3 mg	13%
Selenium	55.6 µg	101%
Sodium	572 mg	38%
Zinc	3.5 mg	32%

Blueberry Chocolate Chip Chia Honey Yogurt
Day 1 – Snack #1

Ingredients	Weight
½ cup plain nonfat yogurt	123 g
1 teaspoon honey	7 g
¼ cup frozen blueberries	58 g
1 tablespoon raisins	9 g
½ tablespoon dark chocolate chips (70-85% cacao)	6 g
2 tablespoons dry oats	10 g
1 teaspoon chia seeds	3 g

Instructions:

Combine all ingredients in a medium bowl.

Energy and Macronutrient Summary

	Amount	Daily Value
Calories	235	12%
Protein	9.9 g	20%
Carbohydrates	40.2 g	
Fiber	4.6 g	16%
Fat	4.8 g	
Omega-3 Fatty Acids	0.6 g	38%

Blueberry Chocolate Chip Chia Honey Yogurt
Vitamin and Mineral Analysis

Vitamins

	Amount	Daily Value
Vitamin A (as Retinol Equivalent Activity)	4 µg	0%
Vitamin B1 (Thiamine)	0.1 mg	12%
Vitamin B2 (Riboflavin)	0.3 mg	27%
Vitamin B3 (Niacin)	0.9 mg	6%
Vitamin B5 (Pantothenic Acid)	1.0 mg	21%
Vitamin B6 (Pyridoxine)	0.2 mg	10%
Vitamin B9 (Folate)	24.8 µg	6%
Vitamin B12 (Cobalamin)	0.8 µg	32%
Vitamin C (Ascorbic Acid)	2.8 mg	3%
Vitamin E (Tocopherol)	0.4 mg	3%
Vitamin K (Phylloquinone)	32 µg	27%
Choline	29.5 mg	5%

Minerals

	Amount	Daily Value
Calcium	282.8 mg	22%
Copper	0.2 mg	27%
Iron	2 mg	11%
Magnesium	68.5 mg	16%
Manganese	0.7 mg	30%
Phosphorus	294.1 mg	24%
Potassium	507.3 mg	11%
Selenium	9.6 µg	17%
Sodium	98.8 mg	7%
Zinc	2.0 mg	18%

Black Bean Turkey Salad with Sunflower Seeds
Day 1 – Lunch

Ingredients	Weight
$\frac{1}{8}$ cup lean ground turkey (7% fat)	29 g
½ cup Romaine lettuce	24 g
¼ medium red onion	28 g
6 grape tomatoes	47 g
8 small baby carrots	52 g
2 tablespoons reduced fat feta cheese	19 g
2 tablespoons unsalted dry roasted sunflower seeds	16 g
Dressing of your choice (optional)	

Instructions:

1. Heat turkey in a skillet until fully cooked.
2. Combine turkey with all other ingredients in a large bowl.

Energy and Macronutrient Summary

	Amount	Daily Value
Calories	360.0	18%
Protein	23.5 g	47%
Carbohydrates	37.2 g	
Fiber	13.4 g	48%
Fat	14.4 g	
Omega-3 Fatty Acids	0.3 g	17%

Black Bean Turkey Salad with Sunflower Seeds
Vitamin and Mineral Analysis

Vitamins

	Amount	Daily Value
Vitamin A (as Retinol Equivalent Activity)	650.9 µg	72%
Vitamin B1 (Thiamine)	0.3 mg	29%
Vitamin B2 (Riboflavin)	0.3 mg	25%
Vitamin B3 (Niacin)	5 mg	31%
Vitamin B5 (Pantothenic Acid)	2.1 mg	43%
Vitamin B6 (Pyridoxine)	0.6 mg	35%
Vitamin B9 (Folate)	218.8 µg	55%
Vitamin B12 (Cobalamin)	0.7 µg	31%
Vitamin C (Ascorbic Acid)	13.6 mg	15%
Vitamin E (Tocopherol)	5 mg	33%
Vitamin K (Phylloquinone)	33.9 µg	28%
Choline	84.1 mg	15%

Minerals

	Amount	Daily Value
Calcium	160.8 mg	12%
Copper	0.6 mg	67%
Iron	3.7 mg	21%
Magnesium	96.3 mg	23%
Manganese	1.0 mg	43%
Phosphorus	474.4 mg	38%
Potassium	965.5 mg	21%
Selenium	25.5 µg	46%
Sodium	303.4 mg	20%
Zinc	3.5 mg	32%

Pear with Molasses Walnut Yogurt
Day 1 – Snack #2

Ingredients	Weight
¼ cup plain nonfat yogurt	61 g
½ teaspoon blackstrap molasses	4 g
2 teaspoons chopped walnuts	5 g
1 medium pear	178 g

Instructions:

1. Combine yogurt, molasses, and walnuts in a small bowl.
2. Slice pear and use yogurt mixture as a dip.

Energy and Macronutrient Summary

	Amount	Daily Value
Calories	179.7	9%
Protein	5.1 g	10%
Carbohydrates	34.9 g	
Fiber	6 g	21%
Fat	3.6 g	
Omega-3 Fatty Acids	0.5 g	29%

Pear with Molasses Walnut Yogurt
Vitamin and Mineral Analysis

Vitamins

	Amount	Daily Value
Vitamin A (as Retinol Equivalent Activity)	3.6 µg	0%
Vitamin B1 (Thiamine)	0.1 mg	6%
Vitamin B2 (Riboflavin)	0.2 mg	15%
Vitamin B3 (Niacin)	0.5 mg	3%
Vitamin B5 (Pantothenic Acid)	0.5 mg	11%
Vitamin B6 (Pyridoxine)	0.1 mg	9%
Vitamin B9 (Folate)	24.7 µg	6%
Vitamin B12 (Cobalamin)	0.4 µg	16%
Vitamin C (Ascorbic Acid)	8.3 mg	9%
Vitamin E (Tocopherol)	0.4 mg	3%
Vitamin K (Phylloquinone)	8.1 µg	7%
Choline	20.8 mg	4%

Minerals

	Amount	Daily Value
Calcium	180.3 mg	14%
Copper	0.3 mg	35%
Iron	0.7 mg	4%
Magnesium	51 mg	12%
Manganese	0.4 mg	16%
Phosphorus	136 mg	11%
Potassium	469.6 mg	10%
Selenium	3.3 µg	6%
Sodium	54.5 mg	4%
Zinc	1.0 mg	9%

Beef Vegetable Lasagna with Whole Grain Bread
Day 1 - Dinner
This recipe makes two servings. Eat second serving for lunch tomorrow.

Ingredients	Weight
½ medium onion	55 g
2 medium carrots	122 g
11½ ounces ground beef, 75% lean	325 g
²/₃ cup vegetable stock	160 g
1 garlic clove	3 g
2 cups tomato purée, sodium-free	500 g
½ cup frozen spinach	95 g
1 cup nonfat cottage cheese	210 g
½ cup shredded mozzarella cheese, part skim milk	56 g
2 thin slices whole wheat bread	48 g

Instructions:

1. Preheat oven to 375°F/190°C.
2. Chop onion and carrots into very small pieces, or shred in a food processor.
3. Cook beef in a skillet over medium heat. Then rinse fat from beef in a strainer.
4. Return beef to skillet. Add vegetable stock and cook until broth has evaporated.
5. Add garlic and vegetables to skillet and cook until vegetables are soft.
6. Add tomato purée to skillet and simmer for 10 minutes.
7. Pour mixture from skillet into a large baking dish.
8. Add spinach and cottage cheese, then stir. Sprinkle shredded cheese on top.
9. Cover dish and bake for 20 minutes or until cheese is golden brown.
10. Serve with toasted bread.
11. Eat one serving tonight and the second serving tomorrow for lunch.

Energy and Macronutrient Summary (one serving)

	Amount	Daily Value
Calories	645.6	32%
Protein	66.8 g	134%
Carbohydrates	53.2 g	
Fiber	10.1 g	36%
Fat	19.6 g	
Omega-3 Fatty Acids	0.2 g	15%

Beef Vegetable Lasagna with Whole Grain Bread
Vitamin and Mineral Analysis (one serving)

Vitamins

	Amount	Daily Value
Vitamin A (as Retinol Equivalent Activity)	929.9 µg	103%
Vitamin B1 (Thiamine)	0.3 mg	28%
Vitamin B2 (Riboflavin)	1.0 mg	73%
Vitamin B3 (Niacin)	13.6 mg	85%
Vitamin B5 (Pantothenic Acid)	3.0 mg	60%
Vitamin B6 (Pyridoxine)	1.1 mg	66%
Vitamin B9 (Folate)	137.7 µg	34%
Vitamin B12 (Cobalamin)	4.6 µg	190%
Vitamin C (Ascorbic Acid)	33.7 mg	37%
Vitamin E (Tocopherol)	8.1 mg	54%
Vitamin K (Phylloquinone)	274.5 µg	229%
Choline	219.7 mg	40%

Minerals

	Amount	Daily Value
Calcium	485.8 mg	37%
Copper	1.0 mg	117%
Iron	10.8 mg	60%
Magnesium	175.7 mg	42%
Manganese	1.5 mg	64%
Phosphorus	845.2 mg	68%
Potassium	2190.1 mg	47%
Selenium	60.6 µg	110%
Sodium	1120.4 mg	75%
Zinc	13.1 mg	119%

Day One Summary

Breakfast
Avocado Toast with Cheesy Coconut Eggs

Snack #1
Blueberry Chocolate Chip Chia Honey Yogurt

Lunch
Black Bean Turkey Salad with Sunflower Seeds

Snack #2
Pear with Molasses Walnut Yogurt

Dinner
Beef Vegetable Lasagna with Whole Grain Bread

Plus 8 cups of tap water throughout the day

Energy and Macronutrient Summary	Amount	Daily Value
Calories	1908.5	95%
Protein	132.7 g	265%
Carbohydrates	194.1 g	
Fiber	39.9 g	142%
Fat	72.1 g	
Omega-3 Fatty Acids	1.8 g	112%

Day One Summary
Vitamin and Mineral Analysis (including tap water)

Vitamins

	Amount	Daily Value
Vitamin A (as Retinol Equivalent Activity)	1781 µg	198%
Vitamin B1 (Thiamine)	1.2 mg	101%
Vitamin B2 (Riboflavin)	2.7 mg	209%
Vitamin B3 (Niacin)	24.4 mg	153%
Vitamin B5 (Pantothenic Acid)	9.6 mg	192%
Vitamin B6 (Pyridoxine)	2.5 mg	145%
Vitamin B9 (Folate)	519.3 µg	130%
Vitamin B12 (Cobalamin)	7.9 µg	330%
Vitamin C (Ascorbic Acid)	117.1 mg	130%
Vitamin E (Tocopherol)	17 mg	114%
Vitamin K (Phylloquinone)	360.8 µg	301%
Choline	677.4 mg	123%

Minerals

	Amount	Daily Value
Calcium	1493.8 mg	115%
Copper	2.7 mg	303%
Iron	20.6 mg	114%
Magnesium	479.7 mg	114%
Manganese	4.7 mg	205%
Phosphorus	2209.2 mg	177%
Potassium	4745.8 mg	101%
Selenium	154.5 µg	281%
Sodium	2225.1 mg	148%
Zinc	23.2 mg	211%

Day Two

Breakfast
Banana Almond Yogurt

Snack #1
Cheesy Egg Muffins

Lunch
Beef Vegetable Lasagna with Whole Grain Bread

Snack #2
Cantaloupe with Sunflower Seeds

Dinner
Black Bean Chicken Feta Salad

Banana Almond Yogurt
Day 2 - Breakfast

Ingredients	Weight
1 medium banana	118 g
½ cup plain yogurt, fat free	123 g
1 teaspoon almond butter, unsalted	5 g
1 tablespoon ground flax seeds	7 g

Instructions:

1. Mash banana in a medium bowl with a fork.
2. Add yogurt, almond butter, and flax seeds to the bowl. Mix together.

Energy and Macronutrient Summary

	Amount	Daily Value
Calories	242	12%
Protein	10.7 g	21%
Carbohydrates	39.4 g	
Fiber	5.5 g	20%
Fat	6.3 g	
Omega-3 Fatty Acids	1.6 g	102%

Banana Almond Yogurt
Vitamin and Mineral Analysis

Vitamins

	Amount	Daily Value
Vitamin A (as Retinol Equivalent Activity)	6.2 µg	1%
Vitamin B1 (Thiamine)	0.2 mg	18%
Vitamin B2 (Riboflavin)	0.4 mg	33%
Vitamin B3 (Niacin)	1.3 mg	8%
Vitamin B5 (Pantothenic Acid)	1.3 mg	25%
Vitamin B6 (Pyridoxine)	0.5 mg	32%
Vitamin B9 (Folate)	47.1 µg	12%
Vitamin B12 (Cobalamin)	0.8 µg	31%
Vitamin C (Ascorbic Acid)	11.4 mg	13%
Vitamin E (Tocopherol)	1.4 mg	9%
Vitamin K (Phylloquinone)	1.1 µg	9%
Choline	38.4 mg	7%

Minerals

	Amount	Daily Value
Calcium	285.9 mg	22%
Copper	0.2 mg	27%
Iron	1 mg	6%
Magnesium	96.6 mg	23%
Manganese	0.6 mg	26%
Phosphorus	289.4 mg	23%
Potassium	860.4 mg	18%
Selenium	7.5 µg	14%
Sodium	98.3 mg	7%
Zinc	1.8 mg	17%

Cheesy Egg Muffins
Day 2 – Snack #1

Ingredients	Weight
1 teaspoon olive oil	5 g
2 tablespoons cream cheese, fat free	31 g
1 large egg	50 g
¼ medium red bell pepper	30 g
3 tablespoons cottage cheese, fat free	39 g
1 teaspoon chia seeds	3 g

Instructions:

1. Preheat oven to 350°F/160°C.
2. Grease a muffin pan with olive oil.
3. Melt cream cheese in a microwave oven for about 1 minute.
4. Add egg to bowl and mix with melted cream cheese until mixture is smooth.
5. Drop egg and cheese mixture into 4 places on the muffin pan.
6. Bake for 5-10 minutes. Chop bell pepper into small pieces while baking.
7. Remove from oven. Top each muffin with cottage cheese, bell pepper, and chia seeds.

Energy and Macronutrient Summary

	Amount	Daily Value
Calories	206.2	10%
Protein	16 g	32%
Carbohydrates	8.6 g	
Fiber	1.7 g	6%
Fat	11.7 g	
Omega-3 Fatty Acids	0.6 g	39%

Cheesy Egg Muffins
Vitamin and Mineral Analysis

Vitamins

	Amount	Daily Value
Vitamin A (as Retinol Equivalent Activity)	208 µg	23%
Vitamin B1 (Thiamine)	0.1 mg	6%
Vitamin B2 (Riboflavin)	0.5 mg	35%
Vitamin B3 (Niacin)	0.6 mg	4%
Vitamin B5 (Pantothenic Acid)	1.2 mg	25%
Vitamin B6 (Pyridoxine)	0.2 mg	12%
Vitamin B9 (Folate)	51.6 µg	13%
Vitamin B12 (Cobalamin)	1.0 µg	43%
Vitamin C (Ascorbic Acid)	38.4 mg	43%
Vitamin E (Tocopherol)	1.7 mg	12%
Vitamin K (Phylloquinone)	26 µg	22%
Choline	177.8 mg	32%

Minerals

	Amount	Daily Value
Calcium	188.4 mg	14%
Copper	0.1 mg	7%
Iron	1.4 mg	8%
Magnesium	31.4 mg	7%
Manganese	0.1 mg	6%
Phosphorus	355.8 mg	28%
Potassium	278.2 mg	6%
Selenium	22.3 µg	40%
Sodium	426.5 mg	28%
Zinc	1.4 mg	13%

Cantaloupe with Sunflower Seeds
Day 2 – Snack #2

Ingredients	Weight
¼ small cantaloupe	110 g
1 tablespoon sunflower seeds, dry roasted, unsalted	31 g

Instructions:

1. Cut ¼ of a small cantaloupe into bite-size pieces and place in bowl.
2. Sprinkle with sunflower seeds.

Energy and Macronutrient Summary

	Amount	Daily Value
Calories	80.6	4%
Protein	2.4 g	5%
Carbohydrates	10.1 g	
Fiber	1.6 g	6%
Fat	4.2 g	
Omega-3 Fatty Acids	0.1 g	3%

Cantaloupe with Sunflower Seeds
Vitamin and Mineral Analysis

Vitamins

	Amount	Daily Value
Vitamin A (as Retinol Equivalent Activity)	169.1 µg	19%
Vitamin B1 (Thiamine)	0 mg	4%
Vitamin B2 (Riboflavin)	0 mg	3%
Vitamin B3 (Niacin)	1.3 mg	8%
Vitamin B5 (Pantothenic Acid)	0.7 mg	13%
Vitamin B6 (Pyridoxine)	0.1 mg	8%
Vitamin B9 (Folate)	40 µg	10%
Vitamin B12 (Cobalamin)	0 µg	0%
Vitamin C (Ascorbic Acid)	36.8 mg	41%
Vitamin E (Tocopherol)	2.1 mg	14%
Vitamin K (Phylloquinone)	2.7 µg	2%
Choline	12 mg	10%

Minerals

	Amount	Daily Value
Calcium	14.6 mg	1%
Copper	0.2 mg	21%
Iron	0.5 mg	3%
Magnesium	22.3 mg	5%
Manganese	0.2 mg	9%
Phosphorus	107.4 mg	9%
Potassium	335 mg	7%
Selenium	6.7 µg	12%
Sodium	16.2 mg	1%
Zinc	0.6 mg	5%

Black Bean Chicken Feta Salad
Day 2 – Dinner

Ingredients	Weight
1 tablespoon olive oil	14 g
1 medium chicken breast, boneless, skinless	120 g
$^1/_3$ cup grapes	50 g
15 arugula leaves	30 g
$^2/_3$ cup black beans, canned, drained, low sodium	115 g
3 tablespoons crumbled feta cheese, reduced fat	28 g
1 tablespoon lemon juice	5 g
Dressing of your choice	
1 cup milk, skim, fat free	245 g

Instructions:

1. Pour olive oil into skillet and heat over medium heat.
2. Cut chicken into bite-sized pieces and cook in skillet until meat is no longer pink.
3. While chicken is cooking, cut grapes in half.
4. Place arugula in medium bowl. Add chicken and other ingredients to bowl.
5. Serve with milk.

Energy and Macronutrient Summary

	Amount	Daily Value
Calories	677.2	34%
Protein	61.9 g	124%
Carbohydrates	53.6 g	
Fiber	13 g	47%
Fat	23.9 g	
Omega-3 Fatty Acids	0.5 g	33%

Black Bean Chicken Feta Salad
Vitamin and Mineral Analysis

Vitamins

	Amount	Daily Value
Vitamin A (as Retinol Equivalent Activity)	320.8 µg	36%
Vitamin B1 (Thiamine)	0.5 mg	45%
Vitamin B2 (Riboflavin)	0.9 mg	66%
Vitamin B3 (Niacin)	16.2 mg	101%
Vitamin B5 (Pantothenic Acid)	2.7 mg	54%
Vitamin B6 (Pyridoxine)	1.1 mg	65%
Vitamin B9 (Folate)	214.4 µg	54%
Vitamin B12 (Cobalamin)	1.9 µg	79%
Vitamin C (Ascorbic Acid)	9.1 mg	10%
Vitamin E (Tocopherol)	2.7 mg	18%
Vitamin K (Phylloquinone)	49.6 µg	41%
Choline	201.3 mg	37%

Minerals

	Amount	Daily Value
Calcium	516.1 mg	40%
Copper	0.4 mg	47%
Iron	4.9 mg	27%
Magnesium	144.2 mg	34%
Manganese	0.8 mg	34%
Phosphorus	765.8 mg	61%
Potassium	1379.9 mg	29%
Selenium	42.9 µg	78%
Sodium	551.9 mg	37%
Zinc	4.4 mg	40%

Day Two Summary

Breakfast
Banana Almond Yogurt

Snack #1
Cheesy Egg Muffins

Lunch
Beef Vegetable Lasagna with Whole Grain Bread

Snack #2
Cantaloupe with Sunflower Seeds

Dinner
Black Bean Chicken Feta Salad

Plus 8 cups of tap water throughout the day

Energy and Macronutrient Summary		
	Amount	Daily Value
Calories	1851.5	93%
Protein	157.7 g	315%
Carbohydrates	161.8 g	
Fiber	31.9 g	114%
Fat	65.7 g	
Omega-3 Fatty Acids	3.1 g	192%

Day Two Summary
Vitamin and Mineral Analysis (including tap water)

Vitamins

	Amount	Daily Value
Vitamin A (as Retinol Equivalent Activity)	134 µg	182%
Vitamin B1 (Thiamine)	1.2 mg	100%
Vitamin B2 (Riboflavin)	2.7 mg	211%
Vitamin B3 (Niacin)	33.1 mg	207%
Vitamin B5 (Pantothenic Acid)	8.9 mg	178%
Vitamin B6 (Pyridoxine)	3.1 mg	1835%
Vitamin B9 (Folate)	490.8 µg	123%
Vitamin B12 (Cobalamin)	8.3 µg	334%
Vitamin C (Ascorbic Acid)	129.4 mg	144%
Vitamin E (Tocopherol)	16 mg	107%
Vitamin K (Phylloquinone)	354 µg	295%
Choline	649.1 mg	118%

Minerals

	Amount	Daily Value
Calcium	1547.7 mg	119%
Copper	2.2 mg	240%
Iron	18.6 mg	103%
Magnesium	489.2 mg	116%
Manganese	3.2 mg	140%
Phosphorus	2263.7 mg	189%
Potassium	5013.6 mg	107%
Selenium	140 µg	255%
Sodium	2289.2 mg	153%
Zinc	21.5 mg	196%

Day Three

Breakfast
Gorgonzola Eggs with Kale

Snack #1
Blackberry Chocolate Smoothie

Lunch
Avocado Tuna Salad with Pumpkin Seeds

Snack #2
Apple with Maple Yogurt

Dinner
Salmon with Zucchini and Black Bean Potato

Gorgonzola Eggs with Kale
Day 3 - Breakfast

Ingredients	Weight
½ tablespoon olive oil	7 g
¼ cup frozen kale, chopped	33 g
2 large eggs	100 g
2 tablespoons Gorgonzola cheese, crumbled	17 g
$^1/_{16}$ teaspoon Himalayan sea salt	
1 slice whole wheat bread, thin-sliced	24 g
1 teaspoon almond butter, unsalted	5 g

Instructions:

1. Pour olive oil into skillet and heat over medium-high heat.
2. Sauté kale for 3-4 minutes.
3. Whisk eggs in a small bowl, then add cheese and salt and mix together.
4. Pour egg mixture into skillet and cook over medium heat until eggs are done.
5. Toast bread and spread almond butter on top.

Energy and Macronutrient Summary

	Amount	Daily Value
Calories	378	19%
Protein	21.2 g	42%
Carbohydrates	14.4 g	
Fiber	2.6 g	9%
Fat	26.3 g	
Omega-3 Fatty Acids	0.2 g	15%

Gorgonzola Eggs with Kale
Vitamin and Mineral Analysis

Vitamins

	Amount	Daily Value
Vitamin A (as Retinol Equivalent Activity)	423.5 µg	47%
Vitamin B1 (Thiamine)	0.2 mg	15%
Vitamin B2 (Riboflavin)	0.7 mg	54%
Vitamin B3 (Niacin)	1.7 mg	11%
Vitamin B5 (Pantothenic Acid)	1.9 mg	38%
Vitamin B6 (Pyridoxine)	0.2 mg	14%
Vitamin B9 (Folate)	67.5 µg	17%
Vitamin B12 (Cobalamin)	1.3 µg	55%
Vitamin C (Ascorbic Acid)	8.3 mg	9%
Vitamin E (Tocopherol)	4.2 mg	28%
Vitamin K (Phylloquinone)	297.9 µg	248%
Choline	305.7 mg	56%

Minerals

	Amount	Daily Value
Calcium	242.1 mg	19%
Copper	0.1 mg	15%
Iron	2.8 mg	15%
Magnesium	51.8 mg	12%
Manganese	0.8 mg	35%
Phosphorus	323.3 mg	26%
Potassium	376.2 mg	8%
Selenium	39.9 µg	72%
Sodium	501 mg	33%
Zinc	2.2 mg	20%

Blackberry Chocolate Smoothie
Day 3 – Snack #1

Ingredients	Weight
¼ dark chocolate bar (70-85% cacao)	10 g
¼ cup skim milk	61 g
1 small banana	101 g
½ cup frozen blackberries, unsweetened	76 g

Instructions:

1. Place chocolate in a small bowl and soften in a microwave for 15-30 seconds.
2. Place other ingredients in a blender. Add the chocolate and blend until smooth.

Energy and Macronutrient Summary

	Amount	Daily Value
Calories	219.1	11%
Protein	4.8 g	10%
Carbohydrates	42.6 g	
Fiber	7.5 g	27%
Fat	5 g	
Omega-3 Fatty Acids	0.1 g	6%

Blackberry Chocolate Smoothie
Vitamin and Mineral Analysis

Vitamins

	Amount	Daily Value
Vitamin A (as Retinol Equivalent Activity)	44.9 µg	5%
Vitamin B1 (Thiamine)	0.1 mg	7%
Vitamin B2 (Riboflavin)	0.2 mg	18%
Vitamin B3 (Niacin)	1.8 mg	11%
Vitamin B5 (Pantothenic Acid)	0.7 mg	14%
Vitamin B6 (Pyridoxine)	0.4 mg	26%
Vitamin B9 (Folate)	50.5 µg	13%
Vitamin B12 (Cobalamin)	0.3 µg	14%
Vitamin C (Ascorbic Acid)	11.1 mg	12%
Vitamin E (Tocopherol)	1.1 mg	7%
Vitamin K (Phylloquinone)	16.3 µg	14%
Choline	27.1 mg	5%

Minerals

	Amount	Daily Value
Calcium	108.8 mg	8%
Copper	0.4 mg	39%
Iron	2.1 mg	12%
Magnesium	73.5 mg	18%
Manganese	1.4 mg	61%
Phosphorus	137.4 mg	11%
Potassium	634.6 mg	14%
Selenium	3.9 µg	7%
Sodium	29.4 mg	2%
Zinc	0.9 mg	8%

Avocado Tuna Salad with Pumpkin Seeds
Day 3 – Lunch

Ingredients	Weight
¼ medium red onion	28 g
¼ medium yellow bell pepper	30 g
½ California avocado	68 g
1 can (5-oz) tuna, water pack, drained	129 g
$^1/_3$ cup black olives, sliced	45 g
5 small baby carrots	32 g
2 tablespoons parmesan cheese	14 g
7 grape tomatoes	55 g
¼ sliced cucumber	54 g
1 teaspoon olive oil	5 g
1 tablespoon lemon juice	5 g
$^1/_{16}$ teaspoon Himalayan sea salt	
1 tablespoon pumpkin seeds, shelled, unsalted	7 g

Instructions:

1. Chop onion and bell pepper into very small pieces. Cut avocado into bite-size pieces. Add to medium-sized bowl.
2. Add all other ingredients to bowl and mix well.
3. Top with pumpkin seeds, olive oil, lemon juice, and salt.

Energy and Macronutrient Summary

	Amount	Daily Value
Calories	467	23%
Protein	35.6 g	71%
Carbohydrates	22.2 g	
Fiber	9.4 g	34%
Fat	28.9 g	
Omega-3 Fatty Acids	0.5 g	31%

Avocado Tuna Salad with Pumpkin Seeds
Vitamin and Mineral Analysis

Vitamins

	Amount	Daily Value
Vitamin A (as Retinol Equivalent Activity)	362.7 µg	40%
Vitamin B1 (Thiamine)	0.2 mg	15%
Vitamin B2 (Riboflavin)	0.3 mg	25%
Vitamin B3 (Niacin)	15.7 mg	98%
Vitamin B5 (Pantothenic Acid)	1.7 mg	33%
Vitamin B6 (Pyridoxine)	0.8 mg	49%
Vitamin B9 (Folate)	102.9 µg	26%
Vitamin B12 (Cobalamin)	3.5 µg	144%
Vitamin C (Ascorbic Acid)	76.5 mg	85%
Vitamin E (Tocopherol)	4 mg	27%
Vitamin K (Phylloquinone)	38.1 µg	32%
Choline	72.1 mg	13%

Minerals

	Amount	Daily Value
Calcium	275.3 mg	21%
Copper	0.5 mg	56%
Iron	5.7 mg	32%
Magnesium	119.5 mg	28%
Manganese	0.7 mg	29%
Phosphorus	449.8 mg	36%
Potassium	1071.5 mg	23%
Selenium	96 µg	175%
Sodium	944 mg	63%
Zinc	2.8 mg	25%

Apple with Maple Yogurt
Day 3 – Snack #2

Ingredients	Weight
3 tablespoons nonfat yogurt	46 g
½ teaspoon maple syrup	3 g
1 small apple	149 g

Instructions:

1. Mix yogurt and maple syrup in a small bowl.
2. Slice apple into several pieces.
3. Dip apple slices in yogurt.

Energy and Macronutrient Summary

	Amount	Daily Value
Calories	111	6%
Protein	3 g	6%
Carbohydrates	26.1 g	
Fiber	3.6 g	13%
Fat	0.3 g	
Omega-3 Fatty Acids	0.0 g	1%

Apple with Maple Yogurt
Vitamin and Mineral Analysis

Vitamins

	Amount	Daily Value
Vitamin A (as Retinol Equivalent Activity)	5 µg	1%
Vitamin B1 (Thiamine)	0.0 mg	4%
Vitamin B2 (Riboflavin)	0.2 mg	14%
Vitamin B3 (Niacin)	0.2 mg	1%
Vitamin B5 (Pantothenic Acid)	0.4 mg	8%
Vitamin B6 (Pyridoxine)	0.1 mg	5%
Vitamin B9 (Folate)	10 µg	22%
Vitamin B12 (Cobalamin)	0.3 µg	12%
Vitamin C (Ascorbic Acid)	7.3 mg	8%
Vitamin E (Tocopherol)	0.3 mg	22%
Vitamin K (Phylloquinone)	3.4 µg	3%
Choline	12.1 mg	2%

Minerals

	Amount	Daily Value
Calcium	103.5 mg	8%
Copper	0.0 mg	5%
Iron	0.2 mg	1%
Magnesium	16.8 mg	4%
Manganese	0.1 mg	6%
Phosphorus	88.7 mg	7%
Potassium	283.1 mg	6%
Selenium	1.7 µg	3%
Sodium	37.3 mg	2%
Zinc	0.5 mg	5%

Salmon with Zucchini and Black Bean Potato
Day 3 - Dinner
This recipe makes two servings. Eat second serving for lunch tomorrow.

Ingredients	Weight
1 large potato	347 g
1 tablespoon olive oil	14 g
10 ounces wild Atlantic salmon	284 g
¼ teaspoon Himalayan sea salt	
1 cup low-sodium black beans, canned, drained	172 g
½ small zucchini	57 g
2 tablespoons nonfat sour cream	28 g
1¼ cup skim milk (for this meal only)	306 g

Instructions:

1. Boil potato for 30-40 minutes.
2. Heat olive oil in a large skillet.
3. Cut salmon into bite-sized pieces and add to skillet. Season salmon with salt.
4. Cook salmon over medium-heat heat for 8-10 minutes or until done.
5. Heat black beans and zucchini (separately) in microwave or over medium heat.
6. Cut potato into pieces and place on plate with salmon and zucchini.
7. Pour olive oil from skillet over potato. Add beans and sour cream on top.
8. Eat one serving tonight with milk. Eat the second serving tomorrow for lunch.

Energy and Macronutrient Summary (one serving)

	Amount	Daily Value
Calories	697	35%
Protein	57.4 g	115%
Carbohydrates	72.9 g	
Fiber	13.9 g	50%
Fat	19.6 g	
Omega-3 Fatty Acids	4.1 g	254%

Salmon with Zucchini and Black Bean Potato
Vitamin and Mineral Analysis (one serving)

Vitamins

	Amount	Daily Value
Vitamin A (as Retinol Equivalent Activity)	221.4 µg	25%
Vitamin B1 (Thiamine)	0.9 mg	73%
Vitamin B2 (Riboflavin)	1.4 mg	111%
Vitamin B3 (Niacin)	17.7 mg	110%
Vitamin B5 (Pantothenic Acid)	5.1 mg	103%
Vitamin B6 (Pyridoxine)	2.1 mg	124%
Vitamin B9 (Folate)	191.7 µg	48%
Vitamin B12 (Cobalamin)	5.9 µg	246%
Vitamin C (Ascorbic Acid)	23.8 mg	26%
Vitamin E (Tocopherol)	6.8 mg	46%
Vitamin K (Phylloquinone)	9.1 µg	46%
Choline	219.6 mg	40%

Minerals

	Amount	Daily Value
Calcium	519.3 mg	40%
Copper	1 mg	111%
Iron	7.6 mg	42%
Magnesium	192.8 mg	46%
Manganese	1.1 mg	48%
Phosphorus	957.9 mg	77%
Potassium	2818.4 mg	60%
Selenium	79.8 µg	145%
Sodium	374.6 mg	25%
Zinc	4.9 mg	45%

Day Three Summary

Breakfast
Gorgonzola Eggs with Kale

Snack #1
Blackberry Chocolate Smoothie

Lunch
Avocado Tuna Salad with Pumpkin Seeds

Snack #2
Apple with Maple Yogurt

Dinner
Salmon with Zucchini and Black Bean Potato

Plus 8 cups of tap water throughout the day

Energy and Macronutrient Summary	Amount	Daily Value
Calories	1872.2	94%
Protein	122.1 g	244%
Carbohydrates	178.3 g	
Fiber	37 g	132%
Fat	80.1 g	
Omega-3 Fatty Acids	4.9 g	307%

Day Three Summary
Vitamin and Mineral Analysis (including tap water)

Vitamins

	Amount	Daily Value
Vitamin A (as Retinol Equivalent Activity)	1057.4 µg	117%
Vitamin B1 (Thiamine)	1.4 mg	115%
Vitamin B2 (Riboflavin)	2.9 mg	222%
Vitamin B3 (Niacin)	37 mg	231%
Vitamin B5 (Pantothenic Acid)	9.8 mg	195%
Vitamin B6 (Pyridoxine)	3.7 mg	218%
Vitamin B9 (Folate)	422.5 µg	106%
Vitamin B12 (Cobalamin)	11.3 µg	470%
Vitamin C (Ascorbic Acid)	127 mg	141%
Vitamin E (Tocopherol)	16.5 mg	110%
Vitamin K (Phylloquinone)	364.7 µg	304%
Choline	636.6 mg	116%

Minerals

	Amount	Daily Value
Calcium	1306 mg	100%
Copper	2.2 mg	247%
Iron	18.3 mg	102%
Magnesium	473.3 mg	113%
Manganese	4.1 mg	180%
Phosphorus	1957.2 mg	157%
Potassium	5183.8 mg	110%
Selenium	221.2 µg	402%
Sodium	1962.1 mg	131%
Zinc	11.5 mg	105%

Day Four

Breakfast
Tomato Feta Eggs with Toast

Snack #1
Chia Cottage Cheese with Figs

Lunch
Salmon with Zucchini and Black Bean Potato

Snack #2
Clams with Spinach and Cheese

Dinner
Chicken Stir Fry

Tomato Feta Eggs with Toast
Day 4 - Breakfast

Ingredients	Weight
½ tablespoon olive oil	7 g
5 grape tomatoes	40 g
2 large eggs	100 g
1/16 teaspoon Himalayan sea salt	
2 tablespoons reduced fat feta cheese, crumbled	19 g
2 slices whole wheat bread, thin-sliced	48 g

Instructions:

1. Pour olive oil into skillet and heat over medium-high heat.
2. Cut grape tomatoes in half or quarters, depending on preference.
3. Sauté tomatoes for 3-4 minutes.
4. Whisk eggs and salt in a small bowl, then add cheese and mix together.
5. Pour egg mixture into skillet and cook over medium heat until eggs are done.
6. Toast two slices of bread, and place on a plate. Spread cooked eggs over toast.

Energy and Macronutrient Summary

	Amount	Daily Value
Calories	384.7	19%
Protein	22.9 g	46%
Carbohydrates	23.9 g	
Fiber	3.4 g	12%
Fat	21.6 g	
Omega-3 Fatty Acids	0.2 g	13%

Tomato Feta Eggs with Toast
Vitamin and Mineral Analysis

Vitamins

	Amount	Daily Value
Vitamin A (as Retinol Equivalent Activity)	249.7 µg	28%
Vitamin B1 (Thiamine)	0.3 mg	24%
Vitamin B2 (Riboflavin)	0.7 mg	54%
Vitamin B3 (Niacin)	2.5 mg	16%
Vitamin B5 (Pantothenic Acid)	1.9 mg	37%
Vitamin B6 (Pyridoxine)	0.3 mg	18%
Vitamin B9 (Folate)	73.7 µg	18%
Vitamin B12 (Cobalamin)	1.3 µg	54%
Vitamin C (Ascorbic Acid)	5.5 mg	6%
Vitamin E (Tocopherol)	3.5 mg	24%
Vitamin K (Phylloquinone)	11.6 µg	10%
Choline	311.7 mg	57%

Minerals

	Amount	Daily Value
Calcium	177.2 mg	14%
Copper	0.1 mg	17%
Iron	3 mg	17%
Magnesium	54.5 mg	13%
Manganese	1.1 mg	49%
Phosphorus	329.2 mg	26%
Potassium	373.9 mg	8%
Selenium	44.9 µg	82%
Sodium	647.6 mg	43%
Zinc	2.3 mg	21%

Chia Cottage Cheese with Figs
Day 4 – Snack #1

Ingredients	Weight
3 dried figs	25 g
½ cup nonfat cottage cheese	105 g
2 teaspoons chia seeds	7 g

Instructions:

1. Cut figs into very small pieces.
2. Add figs to cottage cheese and chia seeds in a small bowl.

Energy and Macronutrient Summary		
	Amount	Daily Value
Calories	171.9	9%
Protein	12.8 g	26%
Carbohydrates	25.9 g	
Fiber	4.9 g	17%
Fat	2.7 g	
Omega-3 Fatty Acids	1.2 g	78%

Chia Cottage Cheese with Figs
Vitamin and Mineral Analysis

Vitamins

	Amount	Daily Value
Vitamin A (as Retinol Equivalent Activity)	2.4 µg	0%
Vitamin B1 (Thiamine)	0.1 mg	5%
Vitamin B2 (Riboflavin)	0.3 mg	20%
Vitamin B3 (Niacin)	0.7 mg	5%
Vitamin B5 (Pantothenic Acid)	0.6 mg	12%
Vitamin B6 (Pyridoxine)	0.1 mg	8%
Vitamin B9 (Folate)	15.1 µg	4%
Vitamin B12 (Cobalamin)	0.5 µg	20%
Vitamin C (Ascorbic Acid)	0.4 mg	0%
Vitamin E (Tocopherol)	0.1 mg	1%
Vitamin K (Phylloquinone)	53.5 µg	1%
Choline	27.3 mg	5%

Minerals

	Amount	Daily Value
Calcium	175 mg	13%
Copper	0.2 mg	19%
Iron	1.8 mg	10%
Magnesium	55.9 mg	13%
Manganese	0.3 mg	15%
Phosphorus	276.5 mg	22%
Potassium	342.3 mg	7%
Selenium	13.9 µg	25%
Sodium	394.2 mg	26%
Zinc	1 mg	9%

Clams with Spinach and Cheese
Day 4 – Snack #2

Ingredients	Weight
¼ cup frozen spinach	48 g
1 can (6½ oz) of clams, drained	83 g
¼ cup shredded mozzarella cheese, part skim milk	28 g

Instructions:

1. Defrost spinach in a microwave oven.
2. Place drained clams on a plate and mix with cheese and spinach.
3. Place plate in microwave oven and cook until cheese is melted.

Energy and Macronutrient Summary

	Amount	Daily Value
Calories	171.9	9%
Protein	12.8 g	26%
Carbohydrates	25.9 g	
Fiber	4.9 g	17%
Fat	2.7 g	
Omega-3 Fatty Acids	1.2 g	78%

Clams with Spinach and Cheese
Vitamin and Mineral Analysis

Vitamins

	Amount	Daily Value
Vitamin A (as Retinol Equivalent Activity)	2.4 µg	0%
Vitamin B1 (Thiamine)	0.1 mg	5%
Vitamin B2 (Riboflavin)	0.3 mg	20%
Vitamin B3 (Niacin)	0.7 mg	5%
Vitamin B5 (Pantothenic Acid)	0.6 mg	12%
Vitamin B6 (Pyridoxine)	0.1 mg	8%
Vitamin B9 (Folate)	15.1 µg	4%
Vitamin B12 (Cobalamin)	0.5 µg	20%
Vitamin C (Ascorbic Acid)	0.4 mg	0%
Vitamin E (Tocopherol)	0.1 mg	1%
Vitamin K (Phylloquinone)	53.5 µg	1%
Choline	27.3 mg	5%

Minerals

	Amount	Daily Value
Calcium	175 mg	13%
Copper	0.2 mg	19%
Iron	1.8 mg	10%
Magnesium	55.9 mg	13%
Manganese	0.3 mg	15%
Phosphorus	276.5 mg	22%
Potassium	342.3 mg	7%
Selenium	13.9 µg	25%
Sodium	394.2 mg	26%
Zinc	1 mg	9%

Chicken Stir Fry
Day 4 - Dinner
This recipe makes two servings. Eat second serving for lunch tomorrow.

Ingredients	Weight
½ cup brown rice (uncooked)	92 g
2 small chicken breasts, boneless, skinless	210 g
1 teaspoon poultry seasoning	
1 tablespoon olive oil	14 g
½ cup raw mushrooms	50 g
½ small white or yellow onion	30 g
½ medium red bell pepper	60 g
20 small baby carrots	130 g
½ cup raw broccoli	92 g
1 tablespoon soy sauce, low-sodium	16 g
1¼ cup skim milk (with tonight's serving only)	306 g

Instructions:

1. Cook rice according to package instructions.
2. Heat olive oil in a large skillet.
3. Defrost chicken and cut into bite-sized pieces. Cook in a skillet over medium-high heat until chicken is no longer pink. Remove chicken from skillet.
4. Cut veggies into small pieces and cook in skillet over medium-high heat for 7-10 minutes.
5. Add chicken to skillet, lower heat to medium, and cook for 7-10 minutes.
6. Mix chicken and vegetables with cooked rice and soy sauce.
7. Eat one serving tonight with milk. Eat the second serving tomorrow for lunch.

Energy and Macronutrient Summary (one serving)

	Amount	Daily Value
Calories	584.1	29%
Protein	50.3 g	101%
Carbohydrates	64 g	
Fiber	6.1 g	22%
Fat	13.9 g	
Omega-3 Fatty Acids	0.2 g	13%

Chicken Stir Fry
Vitamin and Mineral Analysis (one serving)

Vitamins

	Amount	Daily Value
Vitamin A (as Retinol Equivalent Activity)	810.3 µg	90%
Vitamin B1 (Thiamine)	0.6 mg	48%
Vitamin B2 (Riboflavin)	0.9 mg	73%
Vitamin B3 (Niacin)	18.5 mg	116%
Vitamin B5 (Pantothenic Acid)	3.4 mg	69%
Vitamin B6 (Pyridoxine)	1.3 mg	75%
Vitamin B9 (Folate)	93 µg	23%
Vitamin B12 (Cobalamin)	1.9 µg	79%
Vitamin C (Ascorbic Acid)	62 mg	69%
Vitamin E (Tocopherol)	3.2 mg	21%
Vitamin K (Phylloquinone)	58.2 µg	48%
Choline	168.7 mg	31%

Minerals

	Amount	Daily Value
Calcium	445.8 mg	34%
Copper	0.4 mg	42%
Iron	3 mg	16%
Magnesium	143.8 mg	34%
Manganese	1.7 mg	75%
Phosphorus	773.3 mg	62%
Potassium	1326 mg	28%
Selenium	45.9 µg	83%
Sodium	552.7 mg	37%
Zinc	4.2 mg	38%

Day Four Summary

Breakfast
Tomato Feta Eggs with Toast

Snack #1
Chia Cottage Cheese with Figs

Lunch
Salmon with Zucchini and Black Bean Potato

Snack #2
Clams with Spinach and Cheese

Dinner
Chicken Stir Fry

Plus 8 cups of tap water throughout the day

Energy and Macronutrient Summary		
	Amount	Daily Value
Calories	1951	98%
Protein	161.9 g	324%
Carbohydrates	180.3 g	
Fiber	30 g	107%
Fat	64.9 g	
Omega-3 Fatty Acids	6.1 g	383%

Day Four Summary
Vitamin and Mineral Analysis (including tap water)

Vitamins	Amount	Daily Value
Vitamin A (as Retinol Equivalent Activity)	1573.8 µg	175%
Vitamin B1 (Thiamine)	1.7 mg	143%
Vitamin B2 (Riboflavin)	3 mg	233%
Vitamin B3 (Niacin)	39.9 mg	249%
Vitamin B5 (Pantothenic Acid)	10.3 mg	206%
Vitamin B6 (Pyridoxine)	3.8 mg	224%
Vitamin B9 (Folate)	429.7 µg	107%
Vitamin B12 (Cobalamin)	24 µg	999%
Vitamin C (Ascorbic Acid)	92.7 mg	103%
Vitamin E (Tocopherol)	16.5 mg	110%
Vitamin K (Phylloquinone)	392.5 µg	327%
Choline	784.7 mg	143%

Minerals	Amount	Daily Value
Calcium	1323.3 mg	102%
Copper	2 mg	223%
Iron	18.5 mg	103%
Magnesium	505.7 mg	120%
Manganese	4.8 mg	207%
Phosphorus	2476.7 mg	198%
Potassium	5102.1 mg	109%
Selenium	227.3 µg	413%
Sodium	2242.4 mg	149%
Zinc	13.2 mg	120%

Day Five

Breakfast
Mediterranean Eggs with Almond Butter Toast

Snack #1
Blackberry Oatmeal with Walnuts

Lunch
Chicken Stir Fry

Snack #2
Chia Banana Orange Smoothie

Dinner
Beef Bolognese

Mediterranean Eggs with Almond Butter Toast
Day 5 - Breakfast

Ingredients	Weight
1 teaspoon olive oil	5 g
5 small black olives	16 g
4 grape tomatoes	32 g
¼ cup frozen spinach	48 g
2 large eggs	100 g
2 tablespoons blue cheese	17 g
1 thin slice whole wheat bread	24 g
½ tablespoon unsalted almond butter	8 g

Instructions:

1. Pour olive oil into skillet and heat over medium heat.
2. Cut olives and tomatoes in halves or quarters, depending on preference.
3. Sauté olives, tomatoes, and spinach for 4-5 minutes.
4. Whisk eggs in a small bowl, then add cheese and mix together.
5. Pour egg mixture into skillet and cook over medium heat until eggs are done.
6. Toast bread, and spread almond butter over toast. Serve on the side with eggs.

Energy and Macronutrient Summary

	Amount	Daily Value
Calories	406.9	20%
Protein	23 g	46%
Carbohydrates	17.5 g	
Fiber	4.6 g	16%
Fat	27.8 g	
Omega-3 Fatty Acids	0.2 g	15%

Mediterranean Eggs with Almond Butter Toast
Vitamin and Mineral Analysis

Vitamins

	Amount	Daily Value
Vitamin A (as Retinol Equivalent Activity)	478.7 µg	53%
Vitamin B1 (Thiamine)	0.2 mg	19%
Vitamin B2 (Riboflavin)	0.8 mg	62%
Vitamin B3 (Niacin)	2 mg	12%
Vitamin B5 (Pantothenic Acid)	1.9 mg	39%
Vitamin B6 (Pyridoxine)	0.3 mg	19%
Vitamin B9 (Folate)	138.8 µg	35%
Vitamin B12 (Cobalamin)	1.3 µg	55%
Vitamin C (Ascorbic Acid)	7.2 mg	8%
Vitamin E (Tocopherol)	6.2 mg	41%
Vitamin K (Phylloquinone)	186.9 µg	41%
Choline	321.5 mg	58%

Minerals

	Amount	Daily Value
Calcium	285.4 mg	22%
Copper	0.3 mg	31%
Iron	3.7 mg	20%
Magnesium	94.4 mg	22%
Manganese	1.1 mg	48%
Phosphorus	361 mg	29%
Potassium	533.6 mg	11%
Selenium	42.6 µg	78%
Sodium	583.4 mg	39%
Zinc	2.5 mg	23%

Blackberry Oatmeal with Walnuts
Day 5 – Snack #1

Ingredients	Weight
½ cup oats	41 g
1 cup skim milk	245 g
¾ cup blackberries, frozen or fresh	113 g
1 tablespoon chopped walnuts	7 g

Instructions:

1. Put oats and milk in a small pot. Cook over medium-low heat until oats thicken.
2. Defrost blackberries in microwave, if necessary.
3. Pour oatmeal into a small bowl. Add blackberries and sprinkle walnuts on top.

Energy and Macronutrient Summary

	Amount	Daily Value
Calories	356.8	18%
Protein	16 g	32%
Carbohydrates	58.6 g	
Fiber	10.3 g	37%
Fat	7.9 g	
Omega-3 Fatty Acids	0.8 g	48%

Blackberry Oatmeal with Walnuts
Vitamin and Mineral Analysis

Vitamins

	Amount	Daily Value
Vitamin A (as Retinol Equivalent Activity)	155.9 µg	17%
Vitamin B1 (Thiamine)	0.4 mg	30%
Vitamin B2 (Riboflavin)	0.6 mg	44%
Vitamin B3 (Niacin)	2.1 mg	13%
Vitamin B5 (Pantothenic Acid)	1.5 mg	31%
Vitamin B6 (Pyridoxine)	0.2 mg	14%
Vitamin B9 (Folate)	70.7 µg	18%
Vitamin B12 (Cobalamin)	1.2 µg	51%
Vitamin C (Ascorbic Acid)	3.6 mg	4%
Vitamin E (Tocopherol)	1.6 mg	10%
Vitamin K (Phylloquinone)	23.4 µg	19%
Choline	67.1 mg	12%

Minerals

	Amount	Daily Value
Calcium	359.9 mg	28%
Copper	0.4 mg	49%
Iron	2.9 mg	16%
Magnesium	119.5 mg	28%
Manganese	3.1 mg	136%
Phosphorus	473.7 mg	38%
Potassium	719.7 mg	15%
Selenium	20.2 µg	37%
Sodium	106.6 mg	7%
Zinc	3 mg	27%

Chia Banana Orange Smoothie
Day 5 – Snack #2

Ingredients	Weight
¼ cup plain nonfat yogurt	61 g
1 large banana	136 g
1 medium orange	131 g
1 teaspoon chia seeds	3 g

Instructions:

Combine all ingredients in a blender and blend until smooth.

Energy and Macronutrient Summary		
	Amount	Daily Value
Calories	231.4	12%
Protein	6.7 g	13%
Carbohydrates	52.4 g	
Fiber	7.6 g	27%
Fat	1.6 g	
Omega-3 Fatty Acids	0.6 g	36%

Chia Banana Orange Smoothie
Vitamin and Mineral Analysis

Vitamins

	Amount	Daily Value
Vitamin A (as Retinol Equivalent Activity)	20.3 µg	2%
Vitamin B1 (Thiamine)	0.2 mg	16%
Vitamin B2 (Riboflavin)	0.3 mg	23%
Vitamin B3 (Niacin)	1.5 mg	10%
Vitamin B5 (Pantothenic Acid)	1.2 mg	24%
Vitamin B6 (Pyridoxine)	0.7 mg	38%
Vitamin B9 (Folate)	75.3 µg	19%
Vitamin B12 (Cobalamin)	0.4 µg	16%
Vitamin C (Ascorbic Acid)	82.1 mg	91%
Vitamin E (Tocopherol)	0.5 mg	3%
Vitamin K (Phylloquinone)	22.1 µg	18%
Choline	35.6 mg	6%

Minerals

	Amount	Daily Value
Calcium	199.5 mg	15%
Copper	0.2 mg	22%
Iron	1 mg	6%
Magnesium	73.1 mg	17%
Manganese	0.5 mg	21%
Phosphorus	169.8 mg	14%
Potassium	891.8 mg	19%
Selenium	5.9 µg	11%
Sodium	48.8 mg	3%
Zinc	1 mg	9%

Beef Bolognese
Day 5 - Dinner
This recipe makes two servings. Eat second serving for lunch tomorrow.

Ingredients	Weight
1 medium yellow or white onion	110 g
11 ounces ground beef, 75% lean	312 g
2 garlic cloves	6 g
1 tablespoon oregano	3 g
¼ teaspoon Himalayan sea salt	
1 cup tomato puree, no salt added	250 g
2 tablespoons tomato paste, low sodium	32 g
½ cup tap water	118 g
¼ cup nonfat cream cheese	62 g
1 cup skim milk (only with tonight's serving)	245 g

Instructions:

1. Chop onion into very small pieces.
2. Cook beef in a 10-inch skillet over medium-high heat until brown. Drain and rinse beef.
3. Return beef to skillet. Add onion and garlic and continue to cook over medium-high heat for 4-5 minutes.
4. Reduce heat to low. Add oregano, salt, tomato puree, tomato paste, and water. Stir.
5. Simmer for 45 minutes.
6. Add cream cheese and stir.
7. Eat one serving tonight with milk. Eat the second serving tomorrow for lunch.

Energy and Macronutrient Summary (one serving)

	Amount	Daily Value
Calories	470.1	24%
Protein	54.6 g	109%
Carbohydrates	35.9 g	
Fiber	4.5 g	16%
Fat	12.3 g	
Omega-3 Fatty Acids	0.0 g	1%

Beef Bolognese
Vitamin and Mineral Analysis (one serving)

Vitamins

	Amount	Daily Value
Vitamin A (as Retinol Equivalent Activity)	284.6 µg	32%
Vitamin B1 (Thiamine)	0.2 mg	20%
Vitamin B2 (Riboflavin)	0.9 mg	71%
Vitamin B3 (Niacin)	10.3 mg	65%
Vitamin B5 (Pantothenic Acid)	2.7 mg	54%
Vitamin B6 (Pyridoxine)	0.9 mg	54%
Vitamin B9 (Folate)	61.2 µg	15%
Vitamin B12 (Cobalamin)	5 µg	208%
Vitamin C (Ascorbic Acid)	21.8 mg	24%
Vitamin E (Tocopherol)	3.6 mg	24%
Vitamin K (Phylloquinone)	17.4 µg	24%
Choline	213.3 mg	39%

Minerals

	Amount	Daily Value
Calcium	494 mg	38%
Copper	0.6 mg	69%
Iron	7.7 mg	43%
Magnesium	110.5 mg	26%
Manganese	0.5 mg	21%
Phosphorus	770.2 mg	62%
Potassium	1722.5 mg	37%
Selenium	42.4 µg	77%
Sodium	435.5 mg	30%
Zinc	11.7 mg	106%

Day Five Summary

Breakfast
Mediterranean Eggs with Almond Butter Toast

Snack #1
Blackberry Oatmeal with Walnuts

Lunch
Chicken Stir Fry

Snack #2
Chia Banana Orange Smoothie

Dinner
Beef Bolognese

Plus 8 cups of tap water throughout the day

Energy and Macronutrient Summary	Amount	Daily Value
Calories	1945.2	97%
Protein	140.4 g	281%
Carbohydrates	213.3 g	
Fiber	33.1 g	118%
Fat	63.4 g	
Omega-3 Fatty Acids	1.8 g	114%

Day Five Summary
Vitamin and Mineral Analysis (including tap water)

Vitamins

	Amount	Daily Value
Vitamin A (as Retinol Equivalent Activity)	1563.1 µg	174%
Vitamin B1 (Thiamine)	1.5 mg	121%
Vitamin B2 (Riboflavin)	3 mg	229%
Vitamin B3 (Niacin)	34.2 mg	214%
Vitamin B5 (Pantothenic Acid)	9.7 mg	194%
Vitamin B6 (Pyridoxine)	3.3 mg	193%
Vitamin B9 (Folate)	423.7 µg	106%
Vitamin B12 (Cobalamin)	8.3 µg	345%
Vitamin C (Ascorbic Acid)	176.7 mg	196%
Vitamin E (Tocopherol)	15.1 mg	100%
Vitamin K (Phylloquinone)	308 µg	257%
Choline	758.5 mg	138%

Minerals

	Amount	Daily Value
Calcium	1468.1 mg	113%
Copper	2.1 mg	230%
Iron	18.2 mg	101%
Magnesium	526.5 mg	125%
Manganese	6.9 mg	300%
Phosphorus	2238.9 mg	179%
Potassium	4716.1 mg	100%
Selenium	147.5 µg	268%
Sodium	1692.3 mg	113%
Zinc	21.3 mg	194%

Day Six

Breakfast
Nut-n-Honey Apricot Yogurt

Snack #1
Hard Boiled Eggs with Grapes

Lunch
Beef Bolognese

Snack #2
Chia Banana Strawberry Smoothie

Dinner
Barley, Lentil, and Sweet Potato Soup

Nut-n-Honey Apricot Yogurt
Day 6 – Breakfast

Ingredients	Weight
3 dried apricot halves	11 g
½ cup nonfat plain yogurt	123 g
2 tablespoons dry roasted sunflower seeds, unsalted	16 g
2 tablespoons chopped dry toasted almonds, unsalted	16 g
1 teaspoon honey	7 g

Instructions:

1. Cut dried apricot into very small pieces.
2. Put yogurt in a small bowl. Sprinkle with apricots, sunflower seeds, and almonds.
3. Drizzle honey on top.

Energy and Macronutrient Summary

	Amount	Daily Value
Calories	305.5	15%
Protein	13.9 g	28%
Carbohydrates	29.3 g	
Fiber	4 g	14%
Fat	16.7 g	
Omega-3 Fatty Acids	0.0 g	1%

Nut-n-Honey Apricot Yogurt
Vitamin and Mineral Analysis

Vitamins

	Amount	Daily Value
Vitamin A (as Retinol Equivalent Activity)	22.4 µg	2%
Vitamin B1 (Thiamine)	0.1 mg	7%
Vitamin B2 (Riboflavin)	0.5 mg	41%
Vitamin B3 (Niacin)	2.2 mg	13%
Vitamin B5 (Pantothenic Acid)	2 mg	41%
Vitamin B6 (Pyridoxine)	0.2 mg	14%
Vitamin B9 (Folate)	62.7 µg	16%
Vitamin B12 (Cobalamin)	0.8 µg	31%
Vitamin C (Ascorbic Acid)	1.5 mg	2%
Vitamin E (Tocopherol)	8.5 mg	57%
Vitamin K (Phylloquinone)	1 µg	1%
Choline	37.5 mg	7%

Minerals

	Amount	Daily Value
Calcium	305.3 mg	23%
Copper	0.5 mg	59%
Iron	1.6 mg	9%
Magnesium	92.3 mg	22%
Manganese	0.7 mg	32%
Phosphorus	461.4 mg	37%
Potassium	695.2 mg	15%
Selenium	17.7 µg	32%
Sodium	97.1 mg	6%
Zinc	2.6 mg	24%

Hard Boiled Eggs with Grapes
Day 6 – Snack #1

Ingredients	Weight
2 large eggs	100 g
15 grapes (any color)	74 g

Instructions:

1. Place 2 eggs in a pot of water over high heat.
2. When water begins to boil, remove from heat. Put a lid on the pot for 12 minutes.
3. Place eggs in refrigerator (or freezer) to cool, then serve with grapes.

Energy and Macronutrient Summary

	Amount	Daily Value
Calories	206.1	10%
Protein	13.1 g	26%
Carbohydrates	14.5 g	
Fiber	0.7 g	2%
Fat	10.7 g	
Omega-3 Fatty Acids	0.1 g	5%

Hard Boiled Eggs with Grapes
Vitamin and Mineral Analysis

Vitamins

	Amount	Daily Value
Vitamin A (as Retinol Equivalent Activity)	151.8 µg	17%
Vitamin B1 (Thiamine)	0.1 mg	10%
Vitamin B2 (Riboflavin)	0.6 mg	43%
Vitamin B3 (Niacin)	0.2 mg	1%
Vitamin B5 (Pantothenic Acid)	1.4 mg	29%
Vitamin B6 (Pyridoxine)	0.2 mg	11%
Vitamin B9 (Folate)	45.5 µg	11%
Vitamin B12 (Cobalamin)	1.1 µg	46%
Vitamin C (Ascorbic Acid)	2.4 mg	3%
Vitamin E (Tocopherol)	1.3 mg	9%
Vitamin K (Phylloquinone)	11.1 µg	9%
Choline	297.9 mg	54%

Minerals

	Amount	Daily Value
Calcium	57.4 mg	4%
Copper	0.1 mg	12%
Iron	1.5 mg	8%
Magnesium	15.2 mg	4%
Manganese	0.1 mg	3%
Phosphorus	186.8 mg	15%
Potassium	267.3 mg	6%
Selenium	30.9 µg	56%
Sodium	125.5 mg	8%
Zinc	1.1 mg	10%

Chia Banana Strawberry Smoothie
Day 6 – Snack #2

Ingredients	Weight
⅓ cup plain nonfat yogurt	80 g
½ medium banana	59 g
7 medium-sized strawberries	84 g
2 teaspoons chia seeds	7 g

Instructions:

Combine all ingredients in a blender and blend until smooth.

Energy and Macronutrient Summary

	Amount	Daily Value
Calories	158.2	8%
Protein	6.9 g	14%
Carbohydrates	29 g	
Fiber	5.6 g	20%
Fat	2.7 g	
Omega-3 Fatty Acids	1.3 g	82%

Chia Banana Strawberry Smoothie
Vitamin and Mineral Analysis

Vitamins

	Amount	Daily Value
Vitamin A (as Retinol Equivalent Activity)	4.1 µg	0%
Vitamin B1 (Thiamine)	0.1 mg	7%
Vitamin B2 (Riboflavin)	0.3 mg	19%
Vitamin B3 (Niacin)	1.2 mg	8%
Vitamin B5 (Pantothenic Acid)	0.9 mg	17%
Vitamin B6 (Pyridoxine)	0.4 mg	23%
Vitamin B9 (Folate)	45 µg	11%
Vitamin B12 (Cobalamin)	0.5 µg	20%
Vitamin C (Ascorbic Acid)	55.4 mg	62%
Vitamin E (Tocopherol)	0.3 mg	2%
Vitamin K (Phylloquinone)	51.9 µg	43%
Choline	27.3 mg	5%

Minerals

	Amount	Daily Value
Calcium	219.8 mg	17%
Copper	0.2 mg	18%
Iron	1.7 mg	10%
Magnesium	69.4 mg	17%
Manganese	0.7 mg	29%
Phosphorus	218.9 mg	18%
Potassium	572.2 mg	12%
Selenium	7.7 µg	14%
Sodium	64.2 mg	4%
Zinc	1.3 mg	12%

Barley, Lentil, and Sweet Potato Soup
Day 6 - Dinner
This recipe makes two servings. Eat second serving for lunch tomorrow.

Ingredients	Weight
2 medium sweet potatoes	260 g
1 medium white or yellow onion	110 g
4 cups tap water	948 g
2 cups vegetable cooking stock	442 g
2/3 cup dry barley	132 g
2/3 cup pink or red lentils	126 g
30 baby carrots	194 g
2 garlic cloves	6 g
1 tablespoon dried oregano	3 g
1 tablespoon dried thyme	6 g
1 cup skim milk	245 g

Instructions:

1. Chop sweet potato and onion into small pieces.
2. Combine all ingredients in a large stock pot and bring to a boil.
3. When pot begins to boil, lower heat, cover, and simmer for 1 hour.
4. Eat one serving tonight with milk. Eat the second serving tomorrow for lunch.

Energy and Macronutrient Summary (one serving)		
	Amount	Daily Value
Calories	742.5	37%
Protein	34.5 g	69%
Carbohydrates	149.8 g	
Fiber	26.3 g	94%
Fat	3.1 g	
Omega-3 Fatty Acids	0.2 g	15%

Barley, Lentil, and Sweet Potato Soup
Vitamin and Mineral Analysis (one serving)

Vitamins

	Amount	Daily Value
Vitamin A (as Retinol Equivalent Activity)	1917.8 µg	213%
Vitamin B1 (Thiamine)	0.8 mg	69%
Vitamin B2 (Riboflavin)	0.8 mg	62%
Vitamin B3 (Niacin)	6.4 mg	40%
Vitamin B5 (Pantothenic Acid)	2.8 mg	56%
Vitamin B6 (Pyridoxine)	1.1 mg	63%
Vitamin B9 (Folate)	211 µg	53%
Vitamin B12 (Cobalamin)	1.2 µg	51%
Vitamin C (Ascorbic Acid)	17.3 mg	19%
Vitamin E (Tocopherol)	1.7 mg	11%
Vitamin K (Phylloquinone)	74.4 µg	62%
Choline	94.2 mg	17%

Minerals

	Amount	Daily Value
Calcium	538.9 mg	41%
Copper	1.5 mg	167%
Iron	12 mg	67%
Magnesium	184.3 mg	44%
Manganese	2.9 mg	125%
Phosphorus	709 mg	57%
Potassium	1914 mg	41%
Selenium	34.3 µg	62%
Sodium	929.5 mg	62%
Zinc	5.8 mg	53%

Day Six Summary

Breakfast
Nut-n-Honey Apricot Yogurt

Snack #1
Hard Boiled Eggs with Grapes

Lunch
Beef Bolognese

Snack #2
Chia Banana Strawberry Smoothie

Dinner
Barley, Lentil, and Sweet Potato Soup

Plus 8 cups of tap water throughout the day

Energy and Macronutrient Summary		
	Amount	Daily Value
Calories	1799	90%
Protein	114.8 g	230%
Carbohydrates	246.4 g	
Fiber	41.2 g	147%
Fat	45.3 g	
Omega-3 Fatty Acids	1.7 g	104%

Day Six Summary
Vitamin and Mineral Analysis (including tap water)

Vitamins

	Amount	Daily Value
Vitamin A (as Retinol Equivalent Activity)	2231.3 µg	248%
Vitamin B1 (Thiamine)	1.3 mg	105%
Vitamin B2 (Riboflavin)	2.6 mg	202%
Vitamin B3 (Niacin)	20.1 mg	126%
Vitamin B5 (Pantothenic Acid)	9 mg	179%
Vitamin B6 (Pyridoxine)	2.7 mg	159%
Vitamin B9 (Folate)	413.2 µg	103%
Vitamin B12 (Cobalamin)	7.3 µg	306%
Vitamin C (Ascorbic Acid)	98.3 mg	109%
Vitamin E (Tocopherol)	15.4 mg	103%
Vitamin K (Phylloquinone)	155.9 µg	130%
Choline	632 mg	115%

Minerals

	Amount	Daily Value
Calcium	1373.3 mg	106%
Copper	3.1 mg	342%
Iron	24.5 mg	136%
Magnesium	463.6 mg	110%
Manganese	4.8 mg	211%
Phosphorus	2098.9 mg	168%
Potassium	4789 mg	102%
Selenium	125.3 µg	228%
Sodium	1642.7 mg	110%
Zinc	21.7 mg	197%

Day Seven

Breakfast
Chocolate Almond Butter Banana Smoothie

Snack #1
Avocado Egg

Lunch
Barley, Lentil, and Sweet Potato Soup

Snack #2
Orange with Sunflower Seeds

Dinner
Pesto and Cream Chicken with Salad

Chocolate Almond Butter Banana Smoothie
Day 7 – Breakfast

Ingredients	Weight
1 small banana	101 g
2 teaspoons almond butter	10 g
$^2/_3$ cup skim milk	164 g
2 teaspoons cocoa powder, unsweetened	4 g
2 teaspoons chia seeds	7 g
½ tablespoon dark chocolate chips	6 g

Instructions:

1. Combine all ingredients (except chocolate chips) and blend until smooth.
2. Pour smoothie into a glass.
3. Chop or crush chocolate chips and sprinkle on top of smoothie.

Energy and Macronutrient Summary		
	Amount	Daily Value
Calories	286.1	14%
Protein	11.1 g	22%
Carbohydrates	41.1 g	
Fiber	8.2 g	29%
Fat	11.3 g	
Omega-3 Fatty Acids	1.3 g	80%

Chocolate Almond Butter Banana Smoothie
Vitamin and Mineral Analysis

Vitamins

	Amount	Daily Value
Vitamin A (as Retinol Equivalent Activity)	103.6 µg	12%
Vitamin B1 (Thiamine)	0.1 mg	11%
Vitamin B2 (Riboflavin)	0.5 mg	37%
Vitamin B3 (Niacin)	1.7 mg	11%
Vitamin B5 (Pantothenic Acid)	1 mg	21%
Vitamin B6 (Pyridoxine)	0.5 mg	32%
Vitamin B9 (Folate)	39.3 µg	10%
Vitamin B12 (Cobalamin)	0.8 µg	35%
Vitamin C (Ascorbic Acid)	8.9 mg	10%
Vitamin E (Tocopherol)	2.6 mg	18%
Vitamin K (Phylloquinone)	50.7 µg	42%
Choline	46.5 mg	8%

Minerals

	Amount	Daily Value
Calcium	293.5 mg	23%
Copper	0.5 mg	57%
Iron	3.1 mg	17%
Magnesium	134.2 mg	32%
Manganese	1 mg	41%
Phosphorus	346.7 mg	28%
Potassium	824.6 mg	18%
Selenium	11.2 µg	20%
Sodium	73.8 mg	5%
Zinc	2 mg	18%

Avocado Egg
Day 7 – Snack #1

Ingredients	Weight
1 teaspoon olive oil	5 g
1 tablespoon mashed avocado	14 g
1 large egg	50 g

Instructions:

1. Warm olive in small skillet over medium heat.
2. Add mashed avocado to skillet and cook for 1-2 minutes.
3. Whisk egg and add to skillet. Cook until egg is done.

Energy and Macronutrient Summary

	Amount	Daily Value
Calories	145.1	7%
Protein	6.6 g	13%
Carbohydrates	1.8 g	
Fiber	1 g	3%
Fat	12.5 g	
Omega-3 Fatty Acids	0.1 g	6%

Avocado Egg
Vitamin and Mineral Analysis

Vitamins

	Amount	Daily Value
Vitamin A (as Retinol Equivalent Activity)	148.9 µg	27%
Vitamin B1 (Thiamine)	0.0 mg	4%
Vitamin B2 (Riboflavin)	0.3 mg	21%
Vitamin B3 (Niacin)	0.3 mg	2%
Vitamin B5 (Pantothenic Acid)	0.9 mg	18%
Vitamin B6 (Pyridoxine)	0.1 mg	6%
Vitamin B9 (Folate)	34.5 µg	9%
Vitamin B12 (Cobalamin)	0.6 µg	23%
Vitamin C (Ascorbic Acid)	1.2 mg	1%
Vitamin E (Tocopherol)	1.5 mg	10%
Vitamin K (Phylloquinone)	6.1 µg	5%
Choline	148.9 mg	27%

Minerals

	Amount	Daily Value
Calcium	26.9 mg	2%
Copper	0.0 mg	3%
Iron	0.7 mg	4%
Magnesium	9.1 mg	2%
Manganese	0.0 mg	1%
Phosphorus	93.6 mg	7%
Potassium	134 mg	3%
Selenium	15.5 µg	28%
Sodium	63.2 mg	4%
Zinc	0.6 mg	6%

Orange with Sunflower Seeds
Day 7 – Snack #2

Ingredients	Weight
1 small orange	96 g
1½ tablespoons sunflower seeds, dry roasted, unsalted	12 g

Instructions:

Eat orange with sunflower seeds on the side.

Energy and Macronutrient Summary		
	Amount	Daily Value
Calories	115	6%
Protein	3.2 g	6%
Carbohydrates	14.2 g	
Fiber	3.3 g	12%
Fat	6.1 g	
Omega-3 Fatty Acids	0.0 g	1%

Orange with Sunflower Seeds
Vitamin and Mineral Analysis

Vitamins

	Amount	Daily Value
Vitamin A (as Retinol Equivalent Activity)	10.8 µg	11%
Vitamin B1 (Thiamine)	0.1 mg	8%
Vitamin B2 (Riboflavin)	0.1 mg	5%
Vitamin B3 (Niacin)	1.1 mg	7%
Vitamin B5 (Pantothenic Acid)	1.1 mg	22%
Vitamin B6 (Pyridoxine)	0.2 mg	9%
Vitamin B9 (Folate)	57.2 µg	14%
Vitamin B12 (Cobalamin)	0 µg	0%
Vitamin C (Ascorbic Acid)	51.2 mg	57%
Vitamin E (Tocopherol)	3.4 mg	22%
Vitamin K (Phylloquinone)	0.3 µg	0%
Choline	14.7 mg	3%

Minerals

	Amount	Daily Value
Calcium	46.8 mg	4%
Copper	0.3 mg	29%
Iron	0.6 mg	3%
Magnesium	25.1 mg	6%
Manganese	0.3 mg	12%
Phosphorus	152 mg	12%
Potassium	275.8 mg	6%
Selenium	10 µg	18%
Sodium	0.4 mg	0%
Zinc	0.7 mg	6%

Pesto and Cream Chicken with Salad
Day 7 – Dinner

Ingredients	Weight
2 tablespoons brown rice (uncooked)	23 g
1 large chicken breast	135 g
2 tablespoons red pesto sauce (store bought)	31 g
3 tablespoons nonfat cream cheese	47 g
½ cup frozen spinach	78 g
$^2/_3$ cup chopped Romaine lettuce	31 g
4 grape tomatoes	32 g
$^1/_3$ cup raw broccoli	30 g
$^1/_3$ cup raw cauliflower	35 g
4 small baby carrots	26 g
4 small black olives	13 g
1¼ cup skim milk	306 g

Instructions:

1. Preheat oven to 375°F/190°C.
2. Cook rice according to package instructions.
3. Cut chicken into bite-sized pieces. Place into baking dish.
4. Mix pesto and cream cheese until smooth, warming in microwave if necessary.
5. Spread pesto mixture onto chicken.
6. Place baking dish in oven and cook for 35-40 minutes.
7. Serve with salad and milk.

Energy and Macronutrient Summary

	Amount	Daily Value
Calories	677.5	34%
Protein	68.3 g	137%
Carbohydrates	50.2 g	
Fiber	7 g	25%
Fat	22.9 g	
Omega-3 Fatty Acids	0.8 g	53%

Pesto and Cream Chicken with Salad
Vitamin and Mineral Analysis

Vitamins

	Amount	Daily Value
Vitamin A (as Retinol Equivalent Activity)	1207.2 µg	134%
Vitamin B1 (Thiamine)	0.5 mg	46%
Vitamin B2 (Riboflavin)	1.2 mg	90%
Vitamin B3 (Niacin)	20.1 mg	126%
Vitamin B5 (Pantothenic Acid)	3.7 mg	75%
Vitamin B6 (Pyridoxine)	1.4 mg	84%
Vitamin B9 (Folate)	255.5 µg	64%
Vitamin B12 (Cobalamin)	2.5 µg	104%
Vitamin C (Ascorbic Acid)	57.5 mg	64%
Vitamin E (Tocopherol)	5.9 mg	39%
Vitamin K (Phylloquinone)	422.5 µg	352%
Choline	247.2 mg	45%

Minerals

	Amount	Daily Value
Calcium	780.2 mg	60%
Copper	0.5 mg	52%
Iron	5.1 mg	28%
Magnesium	200 mg	48%
Manganese	1.7 mg	72%
Phosphorus	1056.1 mg	84%
Potassium	1758.7 mg	37%
Selenium	56.3 µg	102%
Sodium	1068.8 mg	71%
Zinc	5.3 mg	49%

Day Seven Summary

Breakfast

Chocolate Almond Butter Banana Smoothie

Snack #1

Avocado Egg

Lunch

Barley, Lentil, and Sweet Potato Soup

Snack #2

Orange with Sunflower Seeds

Dinner

Pesto and Cream Chicken with Salad

Plus 8 cups of tap water throughout the day

Energy and Macronutrient Summary

	Amount	Daily Value
Calories	1966.1	98%
Protein	123.8 g	248%
Carbohydrates	257 g	
Fiber	45.8 g	164%
Fat	55.9 g	
Omega-3 Fatty Acids	2.5 g	154%

Day Seven Summary
Vitamin and Mineral Analysis (including tap water)

Vitamins

	Amount	Daily Value
Vitamin A (as Retinol Equivalent Activity)	3315.2 µg	368%
Vitamin B1 (Thiamine)	1.6 mg	136%
Vitamin B2 (Riboflavin)	2.8 mg	216%
Vitamin B3 (Niacin)	29.7 mg	186%
Vitamin B5 (Pantothenic Acid)	9.6 mg	191%
Vitamin B6 (Pyridoxine)	3.3 mg	194%
Vitamin B9 (Folate)	597.4 µg	149%
Vitamin B12 (Cobalamin)	5.1 µg	213%
Vitamin C (Ascorbic Acid)	136.2 mg	151%
Vitamin E (Tocopherol)	15.1 mg	101%
Vitamin K (Phylloquinone)	554.1 µg	462%
Choline	551.4 mg	100%

Minerals

	Amount	Daily Value
Calcium	1743.2 mg	134%
Copper	3 mg	330%
Iron	21.5 mg	119%
Magnesium	571.5 mg	136%
Manganese	5.8 mg	253%
Phosphorus	2357.4 mg	189%
Potassium	4907 mg	104%
Selenium	127.1 µg	231%
Sodium	2211.5 mg	147%
Zinc	14.6 mg	133%